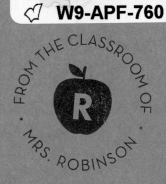

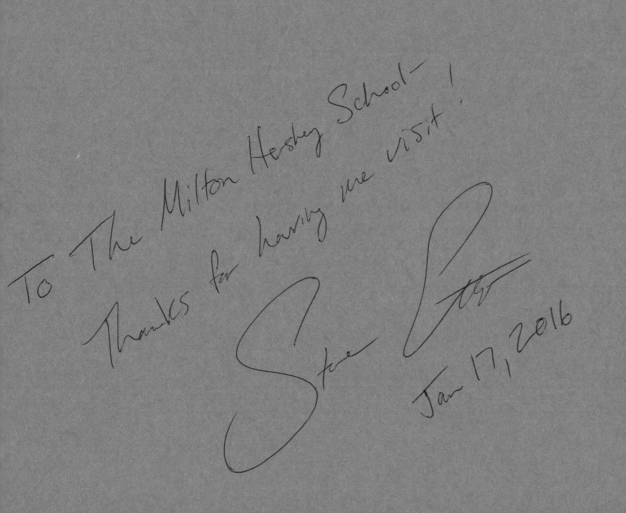

To The Milton Hershey School—
Thanks for having me visit!

Steve P___

Jan 17, 2016

Wallie Exercises

by **Steve Ettinger**, C.S.C.S.

Art by **Pete Proctor**

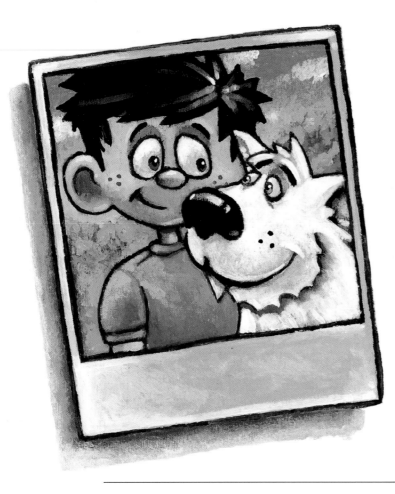

To my four amazing grandparents.
S. E.

For my butter and jelly sandwich.
Love, the Peanut, P. P.

Active Spud Press, New York, NY 10023
www.ActiveSpudPress.com

Text copyright © 2011 by Steve Ettinger
Illustrations copyright © 2011 by Pete Proctor

ISBN: 978-0-9845388-0-5
Library of Congress Control number: 2010936480

10 9 8 7 6 5 4 3 2 1
Printed and bound in the United States of America

Book design by Jill Ronsley, SunEditWrite.com

ActiveSpud PRESS

Disclaimer: The exercises described in this book are
not appropriate for all children and are not intended
to replace the advice of a physician or other healthcare
professional. Please consult with a physician before
your child undertakes any of the exercises.

Wallie was a magnificent mutt,
Calm and cool— not crazy.
Loving and faithful from head to tail—but
Also quite a bit lazy.

While most dogs enjoyed a stroll through the park,
Wallie liked staying indoors.
Other dogs romped around barking their barks
While Wallie mastered his **snores**.

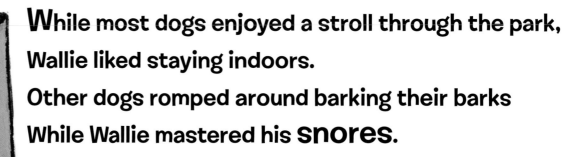

Some hounds performed in fancy dog shows;
Wallie just watched on TV.
Other pups jumped to play fetch with a ball;
Wallie said, "Bring it to me!"

One morning, as always, he woke up late,
But when he went to get dressed,

His **belly** was so big his pants wouldn't fit!
His shirt wouldn't budge past his chest.

Now lazy—and naked—
he plopped down to nap,
"Wallie you need to get up!
Let's find a good place
to get you in shape,"
I said to my pants-less pup.

We drove for a while, miles and miles,
And almost turned back around
When a WIZ and a ZIP took us both by surprise—
Turtles sped by on the ground!

Performing push-ups a few yards away
Were a troop of chimpanzees!
Farther along we spotted giraffes
Doing pull-ups high in the trees . . .

When all of a sudden . . .

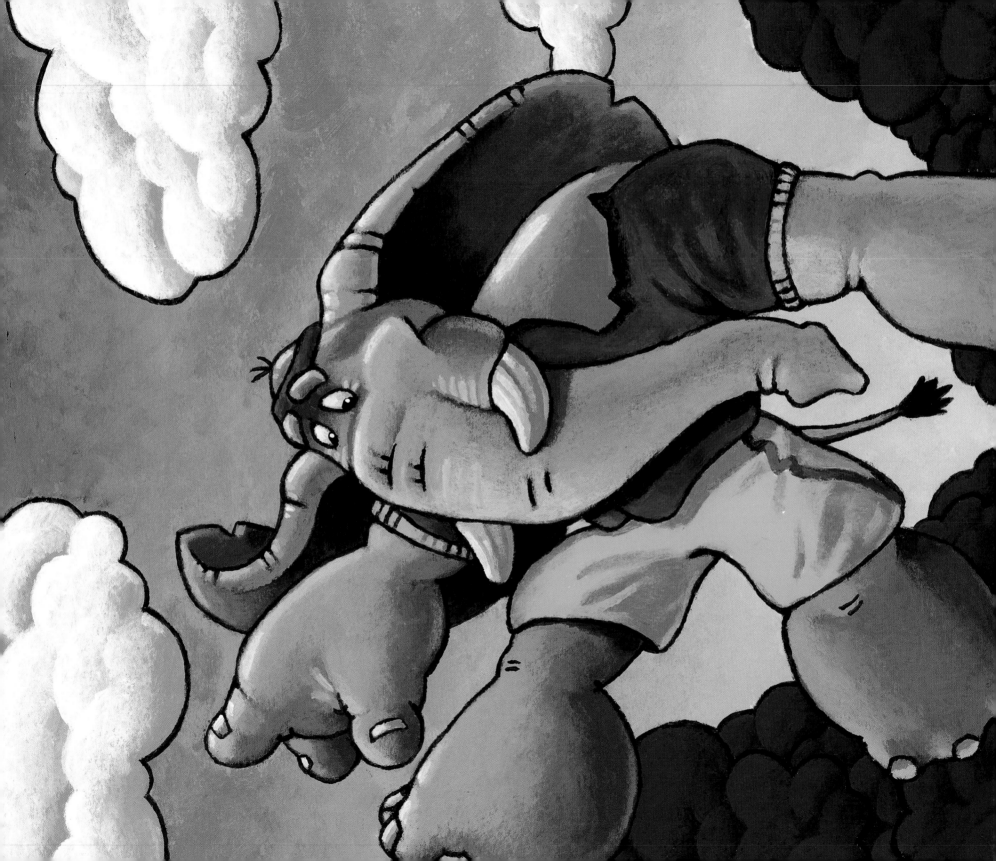

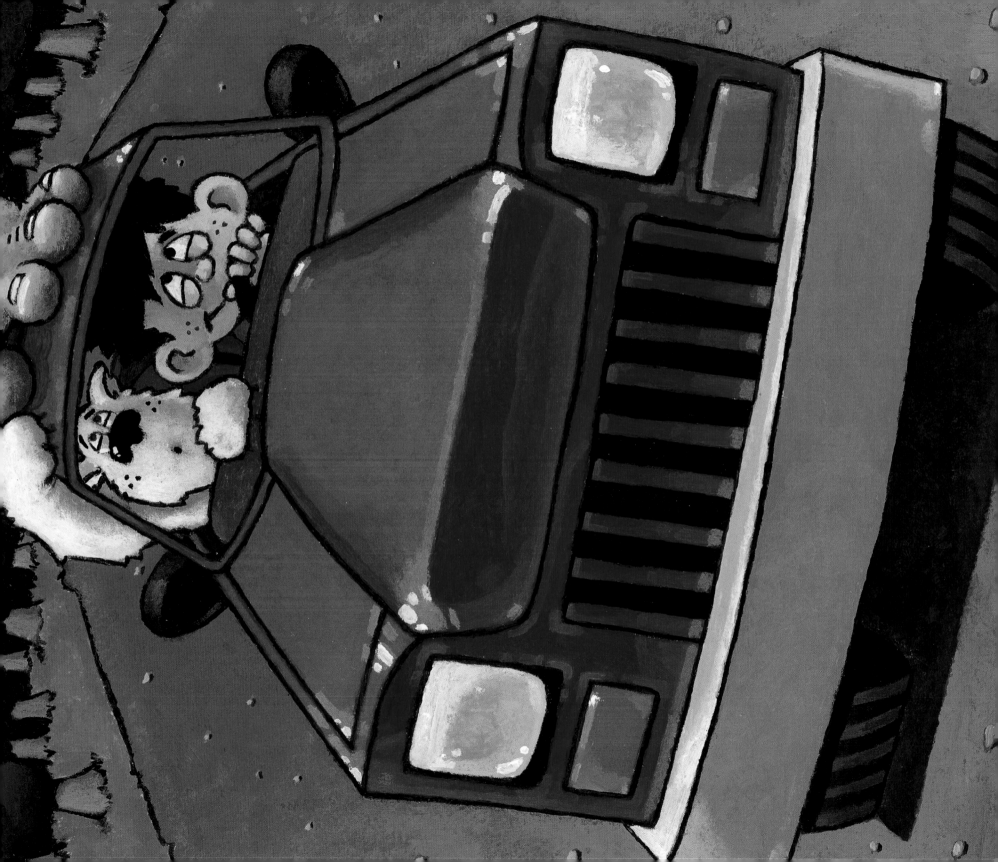

"We're finished!" cried Wallie. "This is the end!
Oh man, he looks mighty mean!
We'll surely be smushed—
he'll eat us for lunch.
I'm gonna be
chubby cuisine!"

The elephant tapped his trunk on the truck,
His tusks turned up in a smile.
"I'm Edwin the Exercise Elephant.
Come, join me for a while.

"You're ready to go, but missing one thing."

He showed us two sweaty sweatbands.

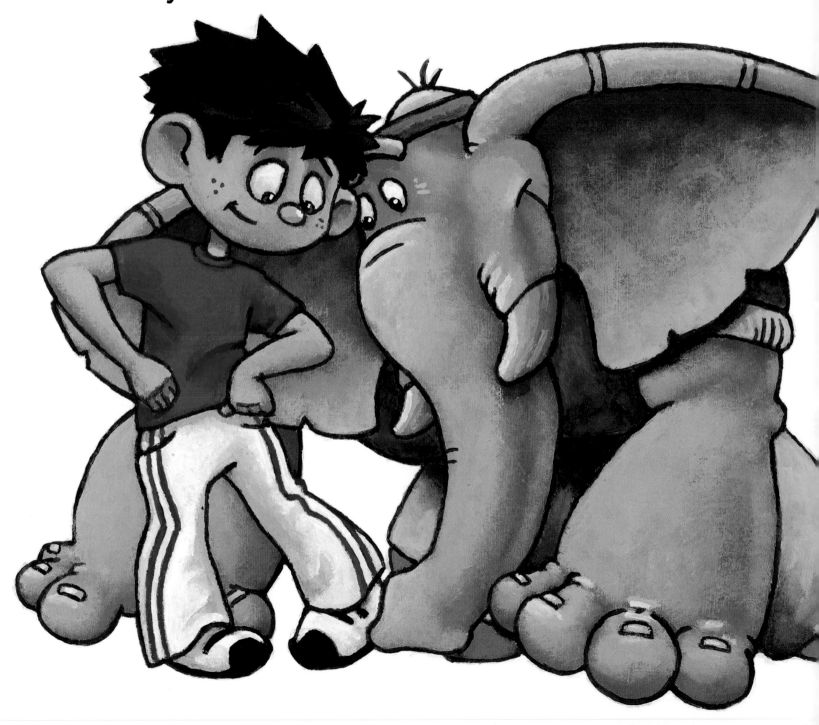

"These are for keeping
the sweat off your trunk
Whenever you do
Trunk Stands."

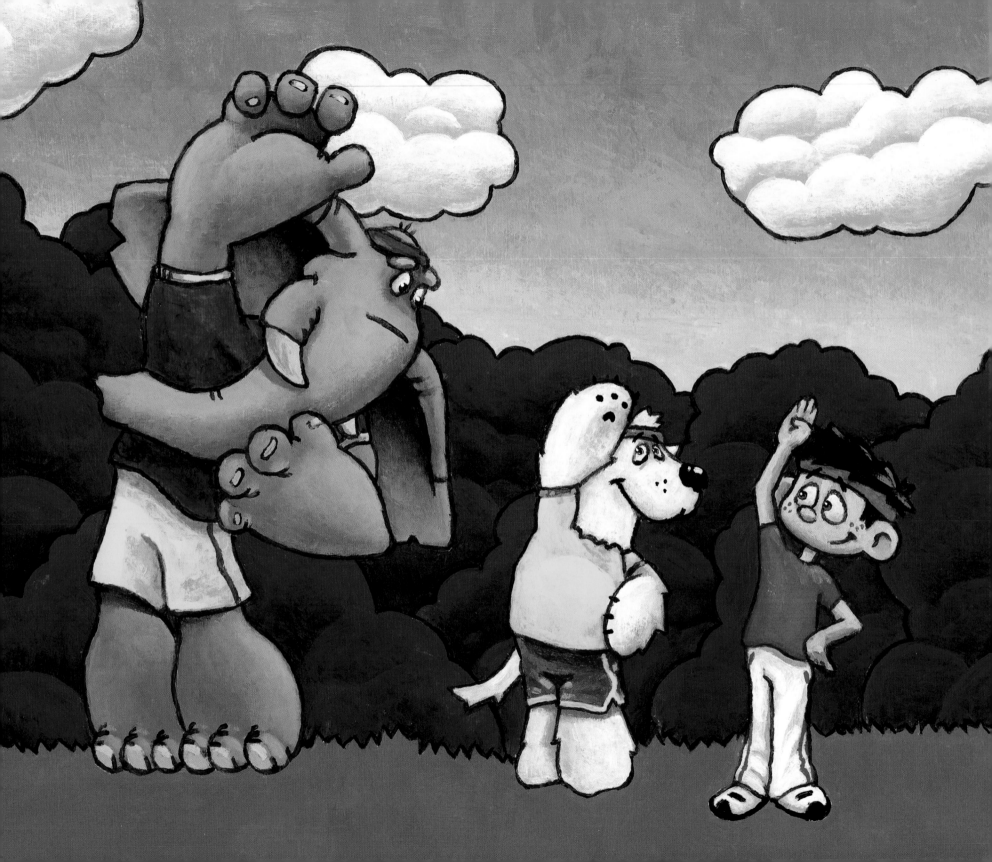

Edwin started us off with a warm-up.

"How easy!" Wallie thought,

But in only a matter of minutes he moaned,

"It's much too doggone hot!"

"**G**ood thinking, Wallie! We need to **hydrate**. Here you go! Gulp it all in.

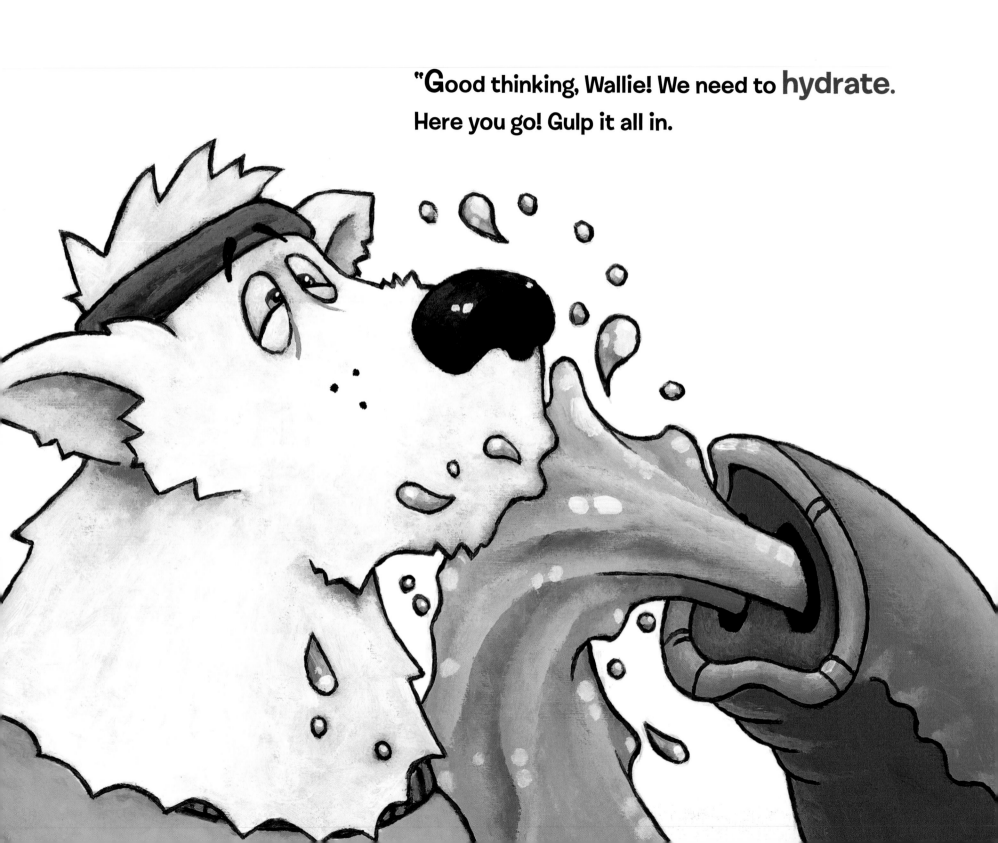

Water keeps us **cool** and ready to move
So we can

jump,

hop

and

spin."

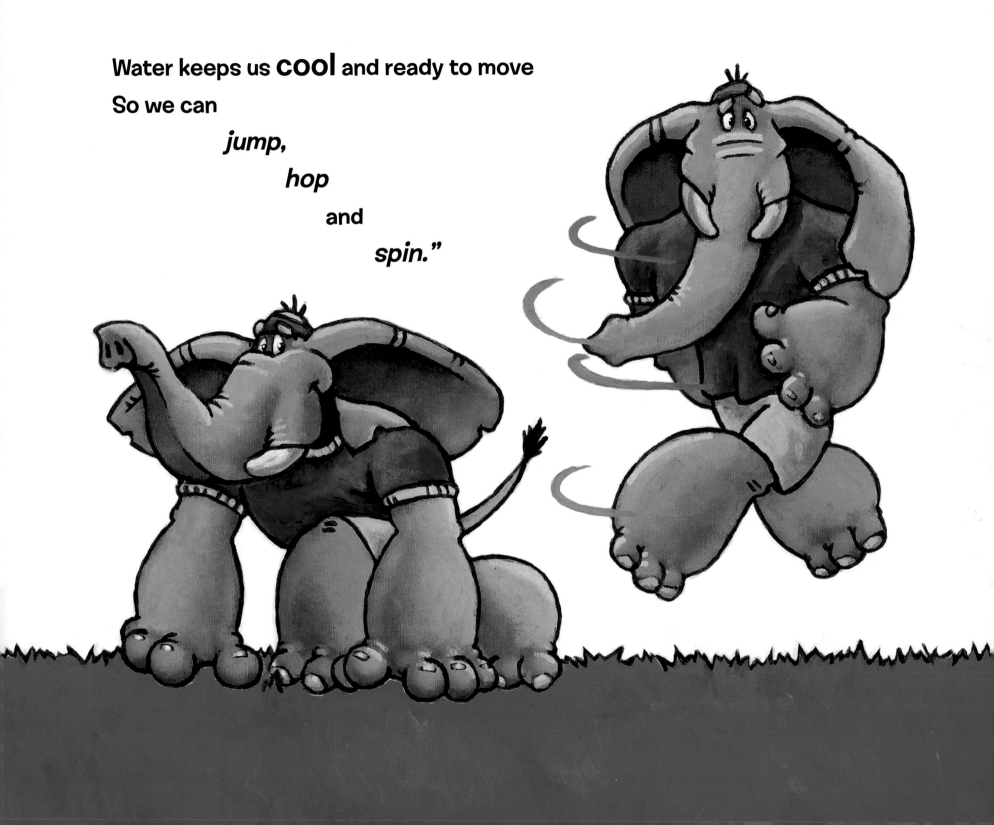

Again Wallie worked without much success,
"Guys, I think I've had enough.
For an out-of-shape pup with a big ole gut,
This stuff is all way too tough."

Edwin convinced him it was worth one more try . . .

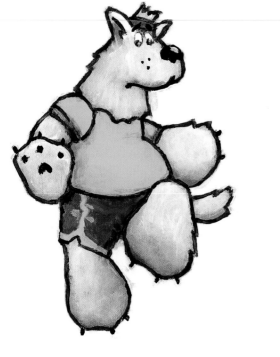

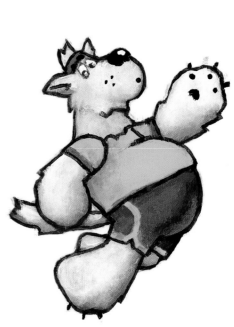

Wallie wobbled and bobbled and skipped,
But just as his snout showed
a hint of a smile,

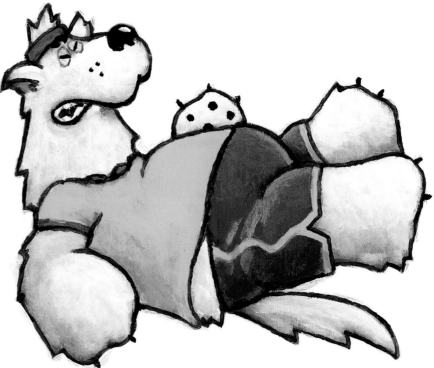

He stepped on his tail and tripped.

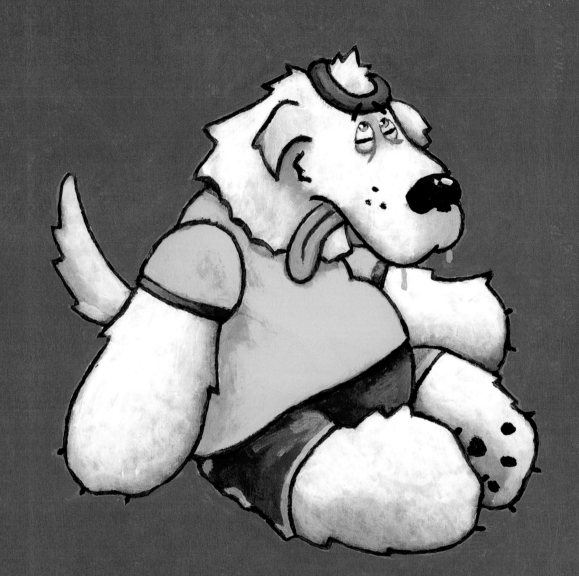

Drool dripped down
from his frown
as he moaned,

"This is as hard as can be.
These exercises are fun for some,
But Edwin, they're not for me."

As Wallie wearily walked away,
Edwin stopped him and said,
"Wallie, you don't have to copy my moves.
Why don't you try yours instead?"

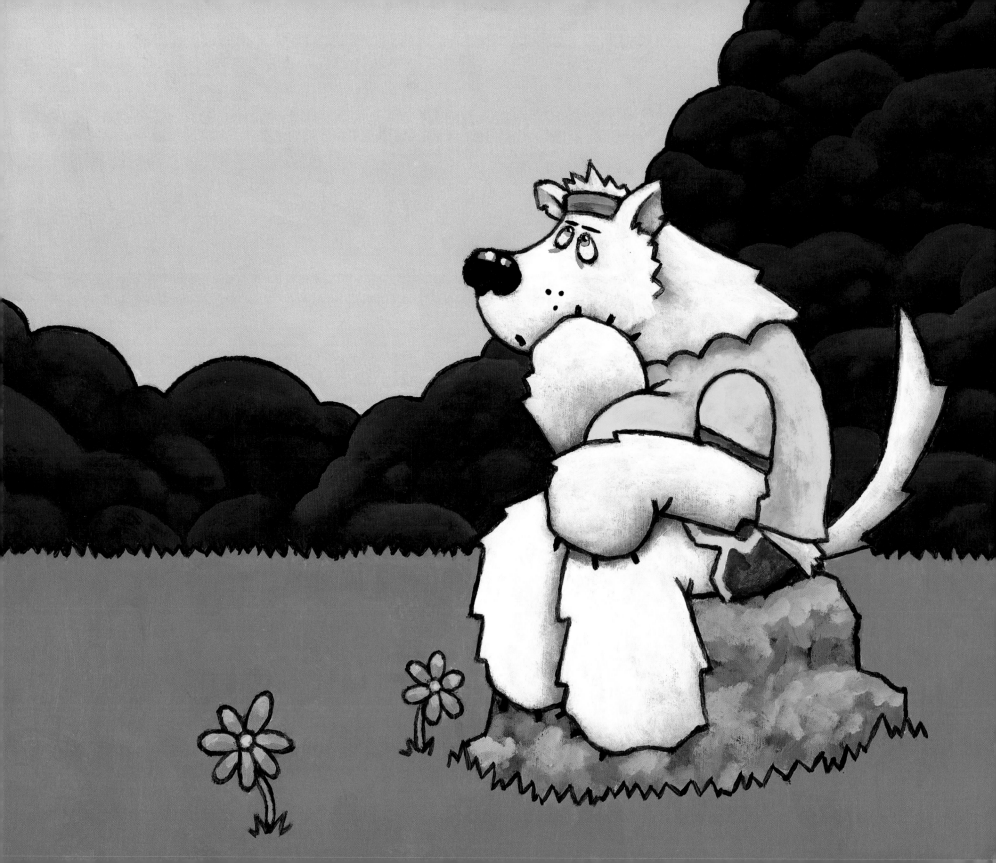

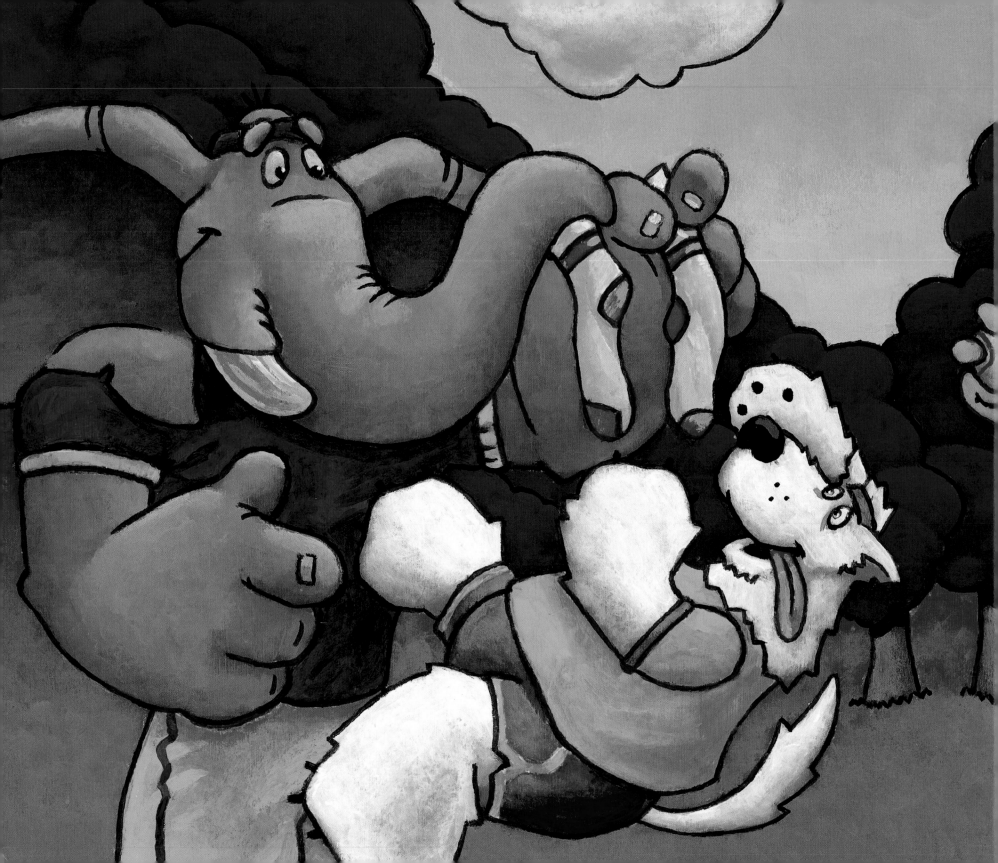

Sweating but smiling,
Wallie wagged his white tail
With glee and joyful surprise . . .

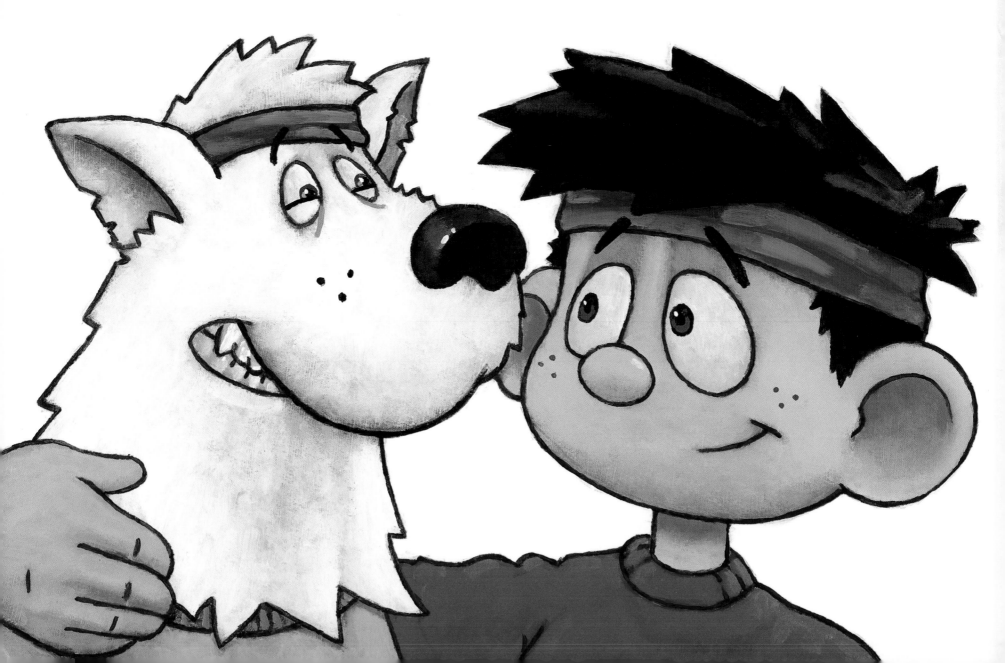

When it finally came time
to leave our new friend,
He shook Wallie's paw and my hand.
As we waved goodbye,
Wallie wondered aloud,

"Hmmm ... How would I do a
trunk stand?"

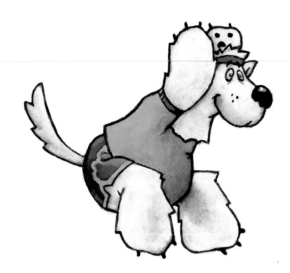

Silly Shark Squat

1. Put your hands (or paws) together on top of your head to make a shark fin.
2. Keeping your head up and back straight, slowly lower your bottom toward the ground.
3. When you're far enough down that you could be sitting in an imaginary chair, stand back up!

Wallie Wiggle Wag Walks and Relay Race

1. To do a Wallie Wiggle Wag Walk, get on your hands and knees.
2. Keep your back straight and head up.
3. Walk forward while shaking your imaginary (or real) tail!

Relay race: Make two or more teams. The first person in each line must race to a designated cone or marker while doing a Wallie Wiggle Wag Walk. When the racers reach the cone, they must do a complete circle around it before returning to their teams and tagging the next person. The first team to have everyone finish, WINS!

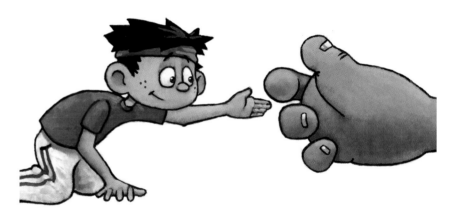

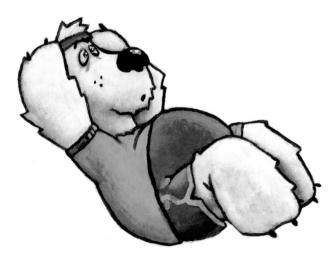

Lazy Tag

1. One person (or more) is the tagger. Everyone else tries to get away from the tagger.
2. If you are tagged, you must lie on your back (like Wallie napping) until a teammate tags you.
3. When this happens you must perform 10 crunches before returning to the game.

EXERCISE can make you healthier, happier, and smarter too! The best part: exercise is **FUN** and there are millions of ways to do it! If you're moving your body, or being **active**, you're probably doing exercise.

> 1. What are some ways that you like to exercise?

WARM-UPS are light exercises done at the beginning of physical activity that help to *warm* your muscles. "Warmed up" muscles perform better and move more easily. This means you can run faster, jump higher, and most importantly, you're less likely to get injured.

> 2. Why do you think it's important that we prepare our bodies for exercise?

HYDRATION is when you drink fluids. When you exercise, you sweat, which is how your body stays cool. By hydrating, you replace some of the water that leaves your body. It's important to hydrate before, during, and after exercise.

> 3. What are some good things to drink when you exercise?

ANSWERS

> 1. Soccer, basketball, tag, jump rope… or you can come up with your own moves!
> 2. We prepare our bodies for exercise so they work better and we don't get hurt.
> 3. Water is one of the best things you can drink during exercise.

For more exercises from "Wallie Exercises"
and more information about keeping kids active and fit, visit

www.ActiveSpudPress.com

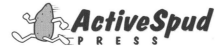

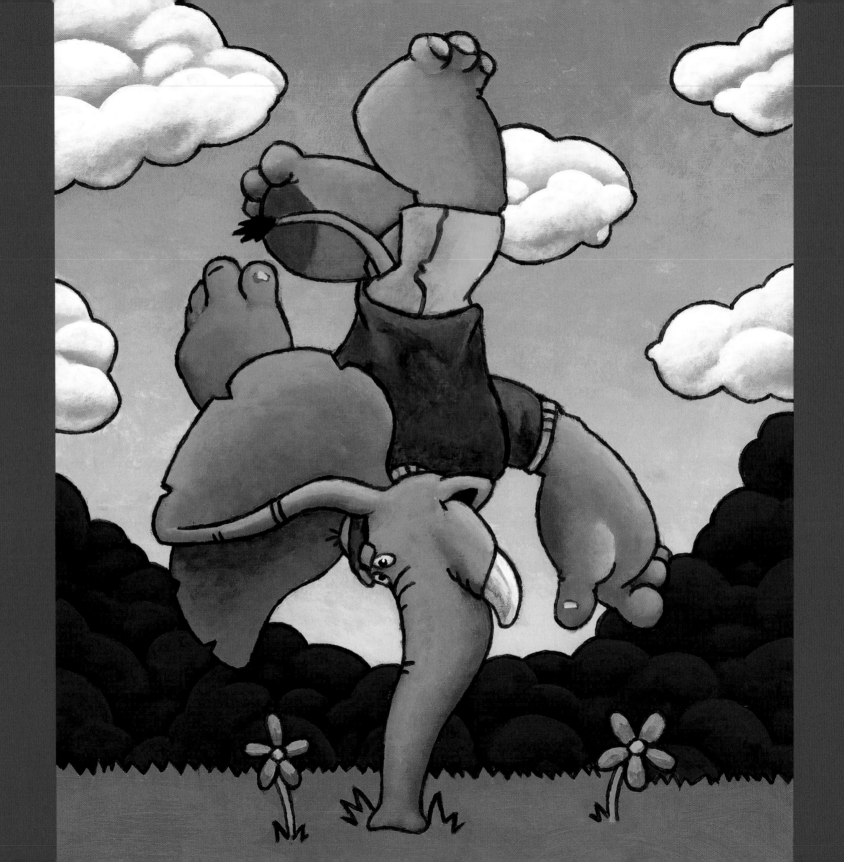